Fast Weight Loss

Cardio Workouts

Table of Contents

These are some of my other books below, and my website is
www.LosingBellyFatMission.com :

https://www.amazon.com/dp/B06XB4WHZX
http://www.amazon.com/dp/B06X9LXBB8
http://www.amazon.com/dp/B06WLK7497
http://www.amazon.com/dp/B06W54JKQN
http://www.amazon.com/dp/B06X6DJ9K3
http://www.amazon.com/dp/B06WGNJ9N3
http://www.amazon.com/dp/B06W549TBD
http://www.amazon.com/dp/B06VTF5DQJ
http://www.amazon.com/dp/B06WRPSBKK
http://www.amazon.com/dp/B06WD194JR
http://www.amazon.com/dp/B06WCZTK7Y
http://www.amazon.com/dp/B06X3QN1HT
http://www.amazon.com/dp/B01N19WBF2
http://www.amazon.com/dp/B01N2AVECA
http://www.amazon.com/dp/B01N4VZIAV
http://www.amazon.com/dp/B00QJJFS1C
http://www.amazon.com/dp/B01EMNO2MW
http://www.amazon.com/dp/B00SSFWCPA
http://www.amazon.com/dp/1520531230
http://www.amazon.com/dp/B01N4V7SR9
http://www.amazon.com/dp/B00SX58DUI
http://www.amazon.com/dp/B010K7YP62
http://www.amazon.com/dp/B012LAYNNQ
http://www.amazon.com/dp/B00RVX3KY2

http://www.amazon.com/dp/B01MR6SWGW
http://www.amazon.com/dp/B00XF6G4HO
http://www.amazon.com/dp/B01F1472N2
http://www.amazon.com/dp/B00PQ0TUPU
http://www.amazon.com/dp/B00PP8OZJ4
http://www.amazon.com/dp/B00QH7DY4Y
http://www.amazon.com/dp/B01052010G
http://www.amazon.com/dp/B00QDHXN7Q
http://www.amazon.com/dp/B00PO0IQIO

Among others.

Easy Ways to Get Rid of Stomach Fat

BREATH	HIP ROLL	NORMAL	BRIDGING
10 Deep Breaths	2 Sets of 10 slow rolls each side - with 20 seconds rest	2 Sets of 10 lifts with 20 seconds rest	1 Set of 10 slow lifts. Hold for 3-5 seconds in upward phase
STANDING ROTATION	**HANDS VIA KNEES**	**SEATED KNEE TUCKS**	**SUPERMANS**
Alternate sides for 30 - 45 seconds	2 Sets of 10 lifts with 20 seconds rest between sets	2 Sets of 6 - 10 lifts with 20 seconds rest between sets	Alternate sides for 45 - 60 seconds

Are you looking for a few easy ways to get rid of stomach fat? Don't really want to go on a diet? Don't really want to spend a lot of time doing cardio exercises? Don't really want to spend a lot of time in the gym? Well, have I got some suggestions for you. Let's start with a basic understanding of what we want to do which is get rid of belly fat.

The reason belly fat is so difficult to get rid of for most people is because they don't understand that you can't spot reduce belly fat. You've got to reduce your overall body fat percentage. This is why doing things like sit ups don't work. Sure, they build muscle but they don't burn enough calories to reduce your overall body fat percentage. So now that we've got that cleared up let's move to nutrition. Don't go on a diet, ever. Diets, by their short term approach to a long term situation, are designed to fail. What you need to do is change your approach toward nutrition.

By simply eliminating soft drinks that contain High Fructose Corn Syrup which converts to fat faster than sucrose you can start shedding the pounds. Drink green tea instead. Studies show that it contains an ingredient which raises your metabolism. Now, let's move to the secret weapon that no one seems to know about. If you really want to increase your metabolism and burn the fat the way to do it is not cardio exercises but doing compound weight lifting exercises. If you spend a half an hour doing things like the clean and jerk, bench press, dead lift and others you will not only be huffing and puffing with exhaustion but you will have effectively thrown your body into a metabolic shock that will burn calories at a higher rate for days after.

Best Cardio Exercises - Get Rid of Excess Fat From Your Body

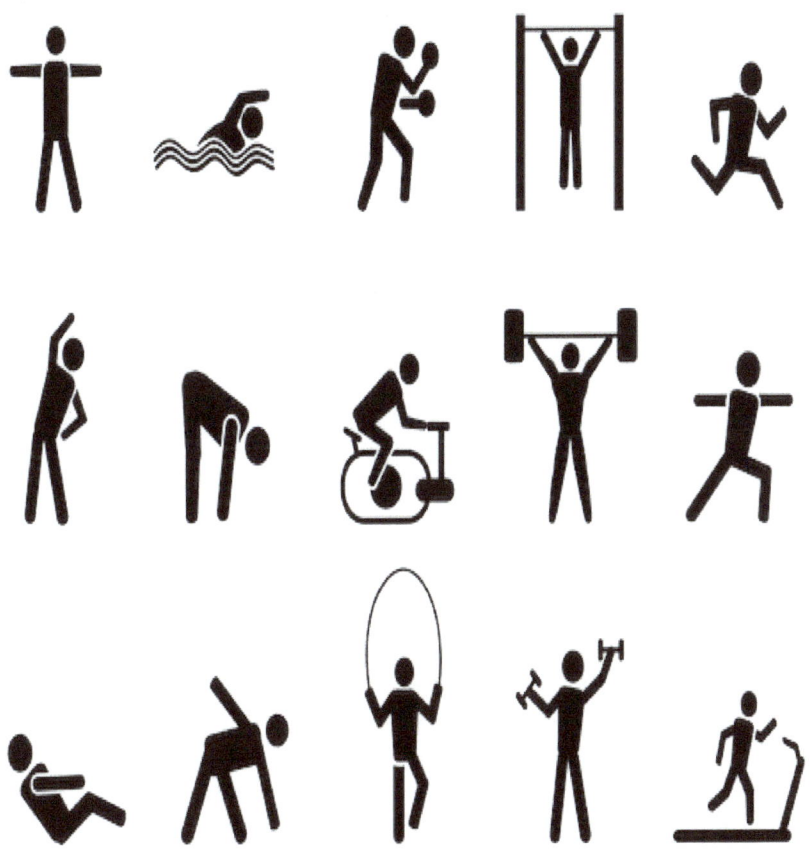

Cardio exercises are best for reducing weight and achieving a slim and sexy body. Cardiovascular exercises not only helps you to get rid of the excess fat from your body what it also helps in strengthening your muscles. Jogging, fast walking, running, swimming and skipping all comes under cardio exercises. This is a best way through which you can burn the ample amount of calories from your body. There are various different types of cardio exercises that you can follow for the different parts of your body. So, now let me tell you about them in great detail.

1.Step

Aerobics Step aerobics is very popular among most women because it really helps you to reduce fat from your legs, hips and thighs. If you are performing it for thirty minutes then you can really burn up to 400 calories.

2. Running

Running is the best cardio exercise that is followed by many people. It is one of the simplest exercises that you can perform without using special equipments and fitness gears. People of all ages can run to reduce their weight. This exercise not only burn calories but is also helps in rejuvenating your mind, body and soul.

3. Bicycling

This is a great outdoor exercise that people of all ages can perform. You can really burn up to 250-500 calories in 30 minutes while bicycling. This exercise really helps in strengthening your leg and thigh muscles.

4. Swimming

Swimming can really help you in strengthening your muscles and burning your fat. Breast stroke is an excellent way through which you can burn up to 400 calories in just thirty minutes. This exercise fully supports your joint that is why there is no fear of getting hurt.

5. Brisk walking

Brisk Walking is also helpful in weight loss. While you are walking you can also include jogging and sprinting to increase the amount of calories that you burn. You can perform this exercise daily in the morning for better results.

6. Rock climbing

Rock climbing is not possible for everyone, but if you are interested in adventurous activities then this exercise is ideal for you. This exercise requires a lot of special equipment and with its help you can burn around 380 calories in half an hour.

7. Skipping

Skipping comes under the category of High Intensity Interval Training and it is a highly effective exercise that can give you great results in just a few days. It provides you a total body workout and can also improve your eye-hand coordination and stamina. Well these are some great cardio exercises that you must follow for better health and stamina.

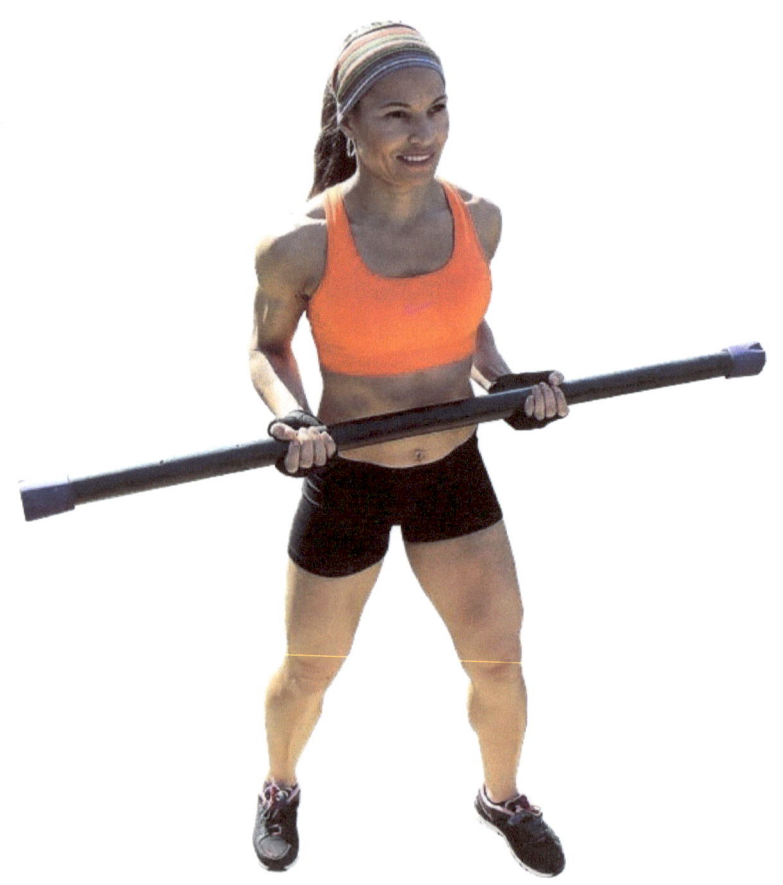

If you want to get an intense cardio workout without having to run a single stride length then you have to incorporate the total body calisthenic of squat thrust into the equation. So what is a calisthenic and what is a squat thrust? Well, to answer both of these questions I will give you a single answer. A calisthenic is a total body exercise performed in a rhythmic systematic way with your own body weight in order to achieve both muscular and cardiovascular strength. A squat thrust is an example of a calisthenic.

Cardio Without Running! If you are going to perform cardio exercises without running and are truly serious about gaining superior muscular and cardiovascular fitness then you have got to engage in the squat thrust calisthenic. This is a sure way for you to increase your perceived level of exertion in order to get the results you want to see the most. So how is a squat thrust done? Well, to begin you will only need your own body weight and a good flat training surface in order to pull it off. Start out by standing with your feet at about shoulder width distance apart in length. From here simply begin this cardio burn by executing 3 different steps. The first step is done by you crouching down in order to place your hands on the ground in front of you. Step 2 is executed by kicking your feet back behind your body extending yourself into an upright push up position. Finally, step 3 is executed by you kicking your feet back up underneath your body in order for you to stand up to complete the drill. All 3 steps constitute a single repetition.

After only performing 10 to 15 of these in a continuous fashion will you understand the meaning of true "cardio" without running. If you were looking for a way to get a hard hitting cardiovascular conditioning workout in without having to run then you just found it. Cardio without a treadmill or an elliptical trainer is good cardio, especially when you are knocking down squat thrusts my friend. Take the time to learn more about this and other great intense workouts by accessing the rest of my articles on the subject for free. Remember that most anyone can train hard, but only the best train smart my friend! Give it a try and see what happens.

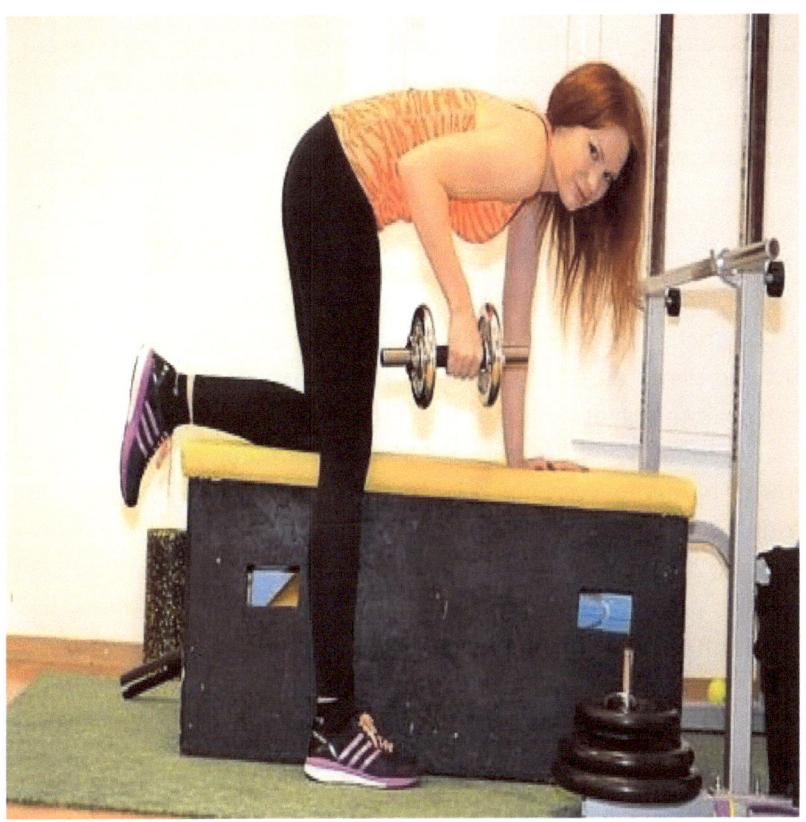

One of the easiest ways of losing belly fat is through cardiovascular exercises. But most people do cardio exercises on their own without consulting a fitness expert. Naturally they end up doing the exercises in the wrong way and fail to get effective results. Here are some guidelines for you to do the cardio exercises in the correct way: Pick the right cardio workout for yourself. Approach a fitness trainer who will suggest you some cardio exercises which will suit your body type. Instead of spending long hours on cardio exercises, do intensive cardio exercises for a short time for effective results. Avoid boredom by having variety in your workout routine. Include at least two types of cardiovascular exercise in your workouts.

High Intensity Interval Cardio (HII Cardio) You can effectively cut down the belly fat by doing HIIT cardio. This kind of workout allows you to change your pace of performance in each workout segment. In one segment you are required to do the exercises really fast while in other segment you can perform at your normal pace. An example of HIIT workout schedule is given below: 2-3 Minutes of medium pace running 1-2 minutes of high pace running 2-3 minutes of fast walking 1 minute of sprinting 2-3 minutes of medium pace running 2-3 minutes of high pace running 2-3 minutes of walking By following such a workout schedule you putting yourself through various levels of intensity which will enable you to burn body fat at a faster rate. But you have to incorporate at least two types of cardio exercises in HIIT workout. Now take a look at some cardio exercises which effectively fights tummy fat. Running By running you get a complete exercise for your entire body. It's a simple exercise which can be done outdoors as well as indoors on a treadmill. Running also provides a great workout for the abs. It activates the muscles in the stomach region and tones them. You can also try sprinting which puts pressure on the abs and helps to burn the excess fat. Wear sports shoes while running to avoid tear and wear of joints and tendons.

Cycling

Cycling is another great workout which effectively burns tummy fat. You can go out cycling with your friends or do it at home on a stationary bike. But you shouldn't workout on a stationary bike that has a back rest since it provides a low intensity workout.

Swimming

Swimming offers a great workout for the entire body and includes movements which activate the major muscles. Swimming is also a fun activity and doesn't feel like a typical workout routine. The different swimming stroke like breast stroke and freestyle targets many muscles of the body and in the process burns fat. You should swim for at least thirty minutes regularly for effective results. Walking When you are brisk walking you tend to breathe faster and suck in more air. The oxygen which you breathe helps to burn your body fat which is essential for staying in shape.

Hiking

Hiking is adventurous and at the same time is a great physical activity for the body. Walking up a hilly region and through a dense forest is pretty challenging which requires a series of movements and in the process you will burn a lot of belly fat.

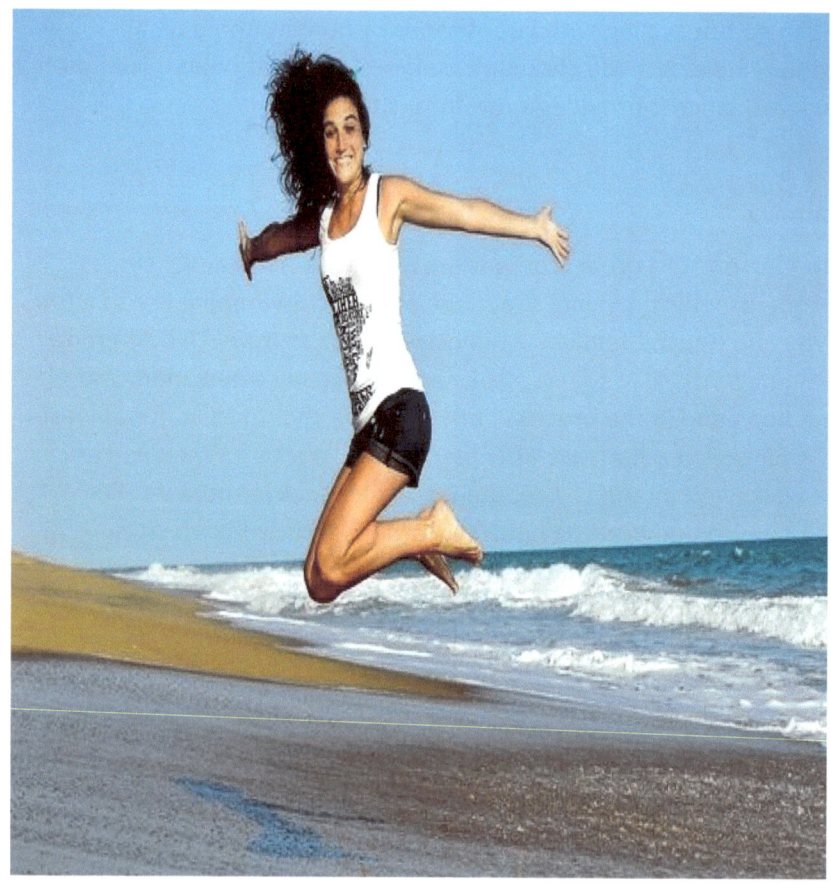

When on vacation you don't want to get out of your workout routine, but you also want to relax and have fun. But how do you stay in shape without your exercise equipment? There are great ways to keep fit when on vacation. First of all it depends on what your normal exercise routine is and where you are during your vacation. But wherever you are, there are ways to keep fit when on vacation.

Do Equipment Free Exercise - Take the chair and do triceps dips every morning - Take the time to do some Yoga. If you have never done Yoga before, check if there is an instructor where you are and give it a try - Take the stairs, do some push ups or lift your kids instead of weights Cardio Exercise When on Vacation - Walk on the beach - to avoid shin splints wear shoes and start with a few minutes at a time.

It might be harder than you think. - Play some sport at the beach with your mates, like beach volleyball, Frisbee or similar - Go hiking or for a bike ride to explore your vacation spot Take some travel friendly workout equipment with you Things like an exercise band or a jump rope fit nicely into your luggage and will help you to keep up your strength and exercise equipment. You can also create your own weights once you have arrived - just keep some water bottles and re-fill them with water.

They make great weights to support your exercise to keep you fit when on vacation. So now there are no more excuses to skip your exercise regime while on vacation. These are easy ways to keep fit when on vacation. And you can also use them as great exercises to do at home!

If you've never had to suffer through the pain of getting rid of man boobs... you don't know how embarrassing they truly are. Man boobs are a medical condition known as gynecomastia... and they are no laughing matter. Man boobs occur when a male has an increased level of estrogen in their body... which in turn causes the mammary glands to swell and enlarge. Weirdly enough, an increase in a person's testosterone level can also cause this condition... excess testosterone can be converted into estrogen by the body.

Gynecomastia happens a lot during puberty... when going through puberty your hormones are often imbalanced and out of whack. This is nothing to worry about because teenagers often grow out of this within a few months.. There are cases when the condition persists.... That's when the problems start! In such cases, getting rid of man boobs takes a little more effort on your part.

What are some of your options?

1. Medication Selective Estrogen Receptor Modulator or SERMs are pills that can be orally ingested by a person who is suffering from gynecomastia. This drug may work either to prevent or stimulate

estrogen production on the body. Some common SERMs are androgens, tamoxifen and raloxifene.

2. Surgery Getting rid of man boobs through the use of surgery may also be an option... There are many surgical procedures like liposuction, a process where all the fats get sucked out of the body. These can scar and are really not good options. Sometimes, man boobs may be caused by obesity. Fats that are stored around the chest contribute to the enlargement of the breasts. This condition is called pseudogynecomastia.

For people who experience this condition, getting rid of man boobs is easier. You simply have to eat right and exercise. Here are some methods that may be effective in getting rid of man boobs:

1.Cardio exercises

Cardio exercises help you burn calories fast. Some recommended cardio exercises are running, biking, rowing, and other activities that keep you active.

2. Strength exercises

These exercises include bench press, weight lifting, and push ups. These are beneficial for toning and firming your chest muscles.

3. Diet

There are a lot of good diet programs that you can subscribe to if you are getting rid of man boobs. Reduce your carbohydrate intake. Avoid foods that are soaked in oil or in butter. Include high protein foods in your diet as protein tends to strengthen the muscles.

How to Decrease Female Body Fat

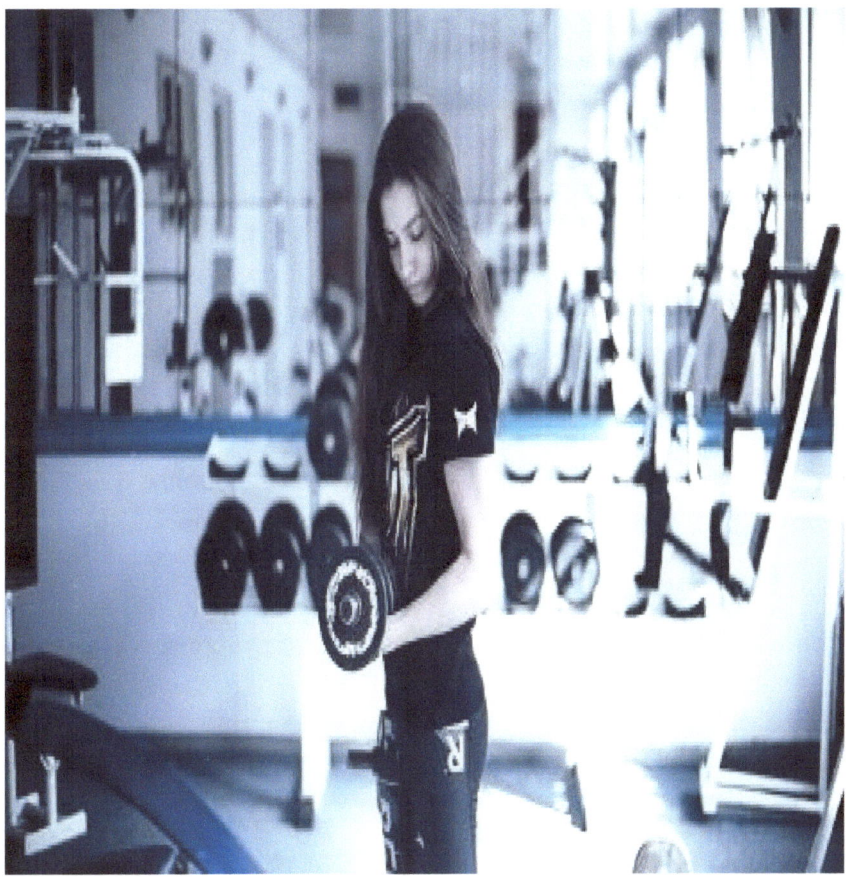

To decrease female body fat is not all that difficult once you know what to do. Unfortunately, most people don't know what to do and spend their time in efforts that won't yield the best results. Let's take a closer look at the situation. You need to burn 3,500 calories to lose a single pound of fat. This is a lot of effort! Some women spend all sorts of time doing sit ups and ab exercises. This is a waste of time for decreasing fat because you can't spot reduce fat. Even if you could, those exercises don't generate nearly enough energy to make a difference.

As a man I have noticed that women tend to gravitate toward the cardio exercises like the treadmill or the Stairmaster while men tend to gravitate toward lifting weights. I think the reason is that by doing those long distance cardio exercises you burn more calories than when you lift weights. This is, in fact true. You burn more calories in a half hour of cardio than you do in a half hour of lifting weights. But, when the exercise if over the fat burning stops as well. Lifting weights is just the opposite. Once the workout is over the fat burning starts because muscle weighs more than fat and the body must work harder and burn more fat.

If you do compound exercises which work multiple muscle groups you will increase your metabolism even more because you throw your body into a state of shock and it will burn calories at a higher rate for days after. Now, I know what you are thinking. I don't want to put on lots of muscle. You won't unless you try. The reason men have bigger muscles is because they are designed to (women aren't) and because they are actively trying to increase their size.

Different Kinds of Cardio Exercises Videos

Living a healthy lifestyle is one of the most important things that every person needs to remember. Risking your health will be one of the worst things that you can ever do, especially with this kind of bipolar weather. Being busy is not an excuse when it comes to exercises, there should always be an allotted time for that. Doing different kinds of exercises will definitely help you become stronger to make you last for the whole busy day. Today, there are tons of ways on how you can do exercise without having to ruin your tight schedule.

There are videos now created for people who would want to do their whole exercise in their own homes. There are cardio exercises videos for a lot of people who wants to burn fat and increase their energy in the easiest ways. You don't need to go to the gym every day since you can do your whole exercise anytime of the day. The good thing about this is that it is way cheaper compared to gym memberships. But before you go into that it is important to understand every cardio exercises to see its effects in the body. The cardio exercises are divided into two first is the slow and steady exercises that generally has a long duration that lasts for 45 minutes to an hour, and the second is the high intensity exercises that has a short duration from 20 to 30 minutes. The latter is said to burn more calories and helps you energetic and stronger the whole day.

Cardio exercises videos have both types of exercises, like for the slow and steady exercise there is the step aerobics. Videos with this kind of exercise uses choreographed dance to keep it more upbeat. There is also what they call zumba, this kind of exercises is all about the latin dance movements. This is now usually seen in health clubs where a lot of people register and there you will see a huge crowd following a certain zumba video for their exercise. For high intensity exercises there are also videos created for this level, and most of the time it is for those who are already used to doing exercises. Some of which are jumping rope videos, this deals with different kinds of exercise and tricks using the jump rope. It may sound simple but it is one of the most effective cardio exercises there is today. It does not only burn fat and calories since it can also help improve -coordination and agility. The famous Tai Bo by Billy Blanks is also one of the many cardio exercises which focuses in cardio kickboxing. It is one of the many favorites of a lot of people since a lot of people have tried had experienced great results.

Other than that aerobics is also a favorite of a lot of people. Every person should always have that desire to live a healthy lifestyle. You can never let yourself die of exhaustion. Start buying exercise videos to help you keep up with your busy and tight schedule.

Easy Cardio Exercises

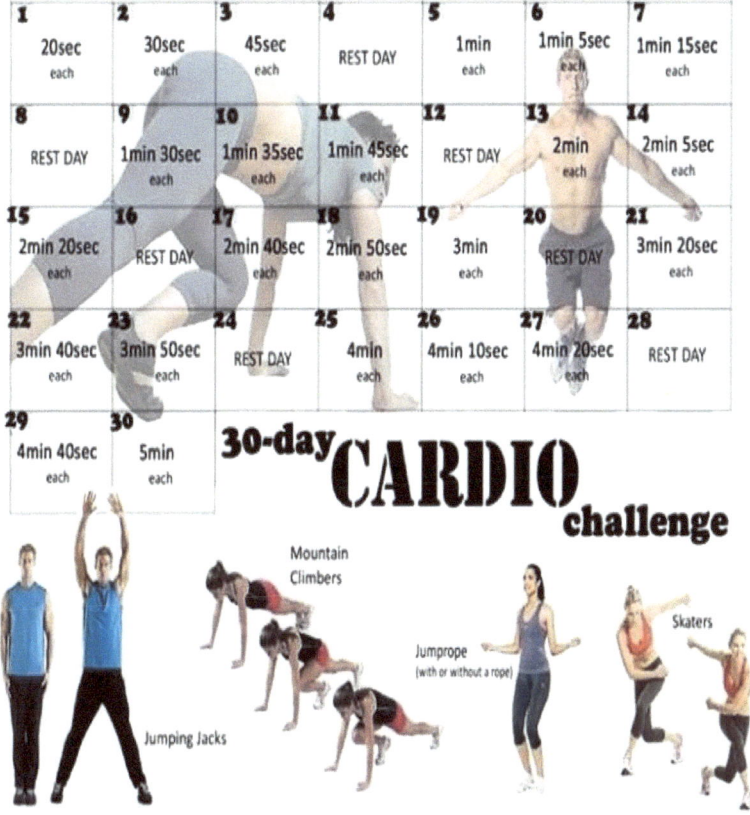

1	2	3	4	5	6	7
20sec each	30sec each	45sec each	REST DAY	1min each	1min 5sec each	1min 15sec each
8	**9**	**10**	**11**	**12**	**13**	**14**
REST DAY	1min 30sec each	1min 35sec each	1min 45sec each	REST DAY	2min each	2min 5sec each
15	**16**	**17**	**18**	**19**	**20**	**21**
2min 20sec each	REST DAY	2min 40sec each	2min 50sec each	3min each	REST DAY	3min 20sec each
22	**23**	**24**	**25**	**26**	**27**	**28**
3min 40sec each	3min 50sec each	REST DAY	4min each	4min 10sec each	4min 20sec each	REST DAY
29	**30**					
4min 40sec each	5min each					

30-day CARDIO challenge

Jumping Jacks

Mountain Climbers

Jumprope (with or without a rope)

Skaters

I'm sure that lots of you don't like the sound of the word cardio. It is a barrier between you and staying fit. Spending most of your time in some boring exercise machines can be agonizing. That is why you have to discover a way on how to make cardio less of a burden for you. Cardio is any activity that raises your heart rate and results to a fat-burning level. In the process, you end up gaining endurance, not to mention the fact that you're losing weight as you do this all. The benefits here are obvious but it is hard work. Well do not fret because there are lots of ways in getting your heart and body active. Below are some ways that will turn your unbearable cardio into an enjoyable routine.

Walking - Humans are meant to walk since prehistoric times. During the Stone Age, men did all of the hunting using their bare feet. So if you are walking for about 45 minutes a day then you are doing yourself a favor. According to studies, many countries are making walking as a part of their culture and people who made walking a part of their everyday life live longer. Well this is no surprise because we all know that our body was designed to move. We are lucky since most of us are required to walk every day, to school, to work or even when going shopping. Brisk walking will give you that fat-burning effect because our heart rate will elevate whilst walking at a standard speed will be advantageous as well as it keeps your body moving.

HIIT - One of the reasons why we all hate to exercise is because we feel like we are distressing ourselves with the long hours we spend on the gym or maybe at home doing some exercise routine. Good thing the HIIT was invented. Here, you can have that body that you've always wanted in 20 minutes or less. The effort that you need to put in this kind of training shouldn't be in its maximum level at all times. Your effort shifts from maximum to moderate depending on the routine that you are performing. Based on studies conducted about cardio, a person can have the same result whether he is spending hours exercising or using the HIIT method. So why would you exhaust yourself when you can do the work in less time? Go for the easier yet effective way so you won't lose your motivation.

These are some of my other books below, and my website is www.LosingBellyFatMission.com :

https://www.amazon.com/dp/B06XB4WHZX
http://www.amazon.com/dp/B06X9LXBB8
http://www.amazon.com/dp/B06WLK7497
http://www.amazon.com/dp/B06W54JKQN
http://www.amazon.com/dp/B06X6DJ9K3
http://www.amazon.com/dp/B06WGNJ9N3
http://www.amazon.com/dp/B06W549TBD
http://www.amazon.com/dp/B06VTF5DQJ
http://www.amazon.com/dp/B06WRPSBKK
http://www.amazon.com/dp/B06WD194JR
http://www.amazon.com/dp/B06WCZTK7Y
http://www.amazon.com/dp/B06X3QN1HT
http://www.amazon.com/dp/B01N19WBF2
http://www.amazon.com/dp/B01N2AVECA
http://www.amazon.com/dp/B01N4VZIAV
http://www.amazon.com/dp/B00QJJFS1C
http://www.amazon.com/dp/B01EMNO2MW
http://www.amazon.com/dp/B00SSFWCPA
http://www.amazon.com/dp/1520531230
http://www.amazon.com/dp/B01N4V7SR9
http://www.amazon.com/dp/B00SX58DUI
http://www.amazon.com/dp/B010K7YP62
http://www.amazon.com/dp/B012LAYNNQ
http://www.amazon.com/dp/B00RVX3KY2
http://www.amazon.com/dp/B01MR6SWGW
http://www.amazon.com/dp/B00XF6G4HO
http://www.amazon.com/dp/B01F1472N2

http://www.amazon.com/dp/B00PQ0TUPU
http://www.amazon.com/dp/B00PP8OZJ4
http://www.amazon.com/dp/B00QH7DY4Y
http://www.amazon.com/dp/B01052010G
http://www.amazon.com/dp/B00QDHXN7Q
http://www.amazon.com/dp/B00PO0IQIO

Among others.